COMPLETE GUIDE TO APPENDICITIS

Navigating Epityphlitis, Understanding Symptoms, Diagnosis, For Expert Guidance On Recognizing Signs, Seeking Help, And Ensuring Speedy Healing

DEHART HAIRSTON

DISCLAIMER

This book's content is only intended for general informative purposes. At the time of writing, the author has taken every precaution to guarantee that the material is correct and current. Nevertheless, the author disclaims all explicit and implicit representations and guarantees about the availability, appropriateness, correctness, completeness, and usefulness of the material on these pages.

Since the author is not a licensed medical practitioner, the material in this book shouldn't be interpreted as medical advice. Before making any modifications to their diet, exercise regimen, or medical treatment, readers are urged to speak with a licensed healthcare provider.

Moreover, the author has no connection to any of the businesses, organizations, or people that are discussed in this book. Any mentions of goods, services, businesses, or people are purely informative and do not indicate endorsement or suggestion.

This book's content is entirely dependent on the author's expertise, study, and comprehension of the topic. Despite having taken reasonable care to offer correct information, the author disclaims all liability for any mistakes or omissions in the material as well as for any losses, harm, or damages resulting from using the information.

It is recommended that readers use their own judgment and discretion when applying the knowledge in this book to their own situations. The use or implementation of any material in this book may result in unfavorable repercussions, directly or indirectly, for which the author assumes no liability.

By reading this book, you agree to release and hold the author harmless from any claims, losses, liabilities, costs, or expenditures resulting from or related to the use of the information you get from it.

ABOUT THIS BOOK

"Appendicitis" is more than simply a book; it is a thorough handbook with the ability to save lives and reduce needless misery. In today's fast-paced society, when health issues may occur suddenly, knowing disorders like appendicitis is essential. This book goes deeply into every facet of the illness, delivering priceless insights that might be the difference between timely treatment and a medical emergency.

Chapter 1 establishes the groundwork by extensively detailing what appendicitis is, its anatomy, causes, and symptoms. With this information, readers may identify warning signals early on, possibly avoiding issues.

Chapter 2 focuses on appendicitis diagnosis, emphasizing the significance of prompt medical attention via physical exams, medical history evaluations, and relevant diagnostics.

Complications are a big worry with appendicitis, as discussed in Chapter 3. Understanding these hazards allows readers to seek medical attention as soon as possible, reducing the risk of perforation and peritonitis.

Chapter 4 discusses treatment alternatives, giving readers a clear grasp of whether they should select surgical removal or antibiotic therapy. Knowing what to anticipate before, during, and after surgery (Chapter 5) is critical for mental preparation and successful recovery.

After surgery, Chapter 6 walks readers through the healing process, including pain management, food issues, and postoperative care. Furthermore, Chapter 7 discusses probable problems following surgery, preparing readers to detect and treat them efficiently.

Prevention is usually preferable to treatment, and Chapter 8 provides helpful insights into lifestyle changes and early symptom detection to avoid appendicitis. The FAQs in Chapter 9 clarify prevalent fallacies and provide light on critical issues concerning the disease.

Finally, Chapter 10 provides a peek into life following an appendectomy, comforting readers about the long-term prognosis and advising them on how to resume regular activities with confidence.

In summary, "Appendicitis" is more than just a book; it's a lifeline for anybody looking to better understand, avoid, or treat this potentially fatal infection. This book is a must-have for any medical practitioner, caregiver, or anybody looking to protect their health.

CHAPTER 1

Understanding Appendicitis

What Is Appendicitis?

Appendicitis is a medical illness characterized by inflammation of the appendix, which is a tiny, finger-shaped pouch found where the small and large intestines meet. This inflammation is often induced by an obstruction, which might be due to feces, a foreign material, or a tumor. When the appendix gets obstructed, germs may thrive within, causing infection and inflammation. If left untreated, appendicitis may lead to a ruptured appendix, which can be fatal.

Anatomy Of The Appendix

The appendix is a tiny organ found on the lower right side of the abdomen. Although its specific function is unknown, it is thought to have a role in the immune system, especially in the early years of life. The appendix connects to the large intestine and has a thin, tube-like shape. Its placement renders it prone to obstructions, which might result in appendicitis.

Causes And Risk Factors

Several variables may influence the development of appendicitis. One frequent cause is appendix obstruction, which may develop from a variety of causes, including solid feces, enlarged lymphoid follicles, parasites, and even malignancies. When the appendix gets obstructed, germs may thrive within, causing infection and inflammation.

Certain risk factors may increase the probability of having appendicitis. This includes:

1. Appendicitis often affects people between the ages of 10 and 30, however, it may occur at any age.

2. Gender: Men are somewhat more likely than women to get appendicitis.

3. Family History: People who have a family history of appendicitis may be more likely to get the illness themselves.

4. Diet: A diet low in fiber and heavy in processed foods may raise the risk of appendicitis by causing constipation and fecal obstructions.

5. Individuals who have had abdominal surgery may be somewhat more likely to develop appendicitis owing to scar tissue buildup.

Signs And Symptoms

Recognizing the symptoms of appendicitis is critical for early diagnosis and treatment. The most prevalent symptoms are:

1. Abdominal Pain: The major symptom of appendicitis is usually abdominal pain that begins at the navel and spreads to the lower right side of the abdomen. Pain may intensify with movement, coughing, or sneezing.

2. Loss of Appetite: Many people with appendicitis lose their appetite and may avoid eating owing to nausea and abdominal pain.

3. Nausea and vomiting are frequent symptoms of appendicitis, and they are commonly accompanied by abdominal pain.

4. Fever: Appendicitis may cause a low-grade fever, particularly if the appendix has burst or become highly inflamed.

5. Other signs of appendicitis include stomach swelling, constipation or diarrhea, and trouble passing gas.

It is crucial to note that the presentation of symptoms varies from person to person, and not everyone with appendicitis will exhibit all of the symptoms mentioned above. If you believe you or someone else has appendicitis, get medical help right once to ensure correct diagnosis and treatment.

CHAPTER 2

Diagnosing Appendicitis

Physical Examination

When diagnosing appendicitis, a comprehensive physical examination is required. The doctor will begin by evaluating vital indicators such as temperature, heart rate, and blood pressure. They will next do a thorough examination of the abdomen. The doctor will gently push on various places of the belly to look for soreness, particularly in the right lower quadrant, where the appendix is situated.

During the physical examination, the physician may also administer the rebound tenderness test. This entails putting pressure on the abdomen and rapidly releasing it. If the pain intensifies when the pressure is removed, this might be an indication of appendicitis. Additionally, the doctor may look for a condition known as Rovsing's sign, in which pushing on the left lower abdomen generates discomfort in the right lower abdomen.

Other indicators that may be assessed during the examination include guarding (muscle tensing), rigidity (abdominal stiffness), and a positive psoas sign.

Medical History Assessment

A thorough medical history review is another critical component in diagnosing appendicitis. The doctor will ask about the patient's symptoms, including when they began, how severe they are, and if they have worsened over time. They will also inquire about any accompanying symptoms, such as nausea, vomiting, gastrointestinal abnormalities, and appetite loss.

The medical history evaluation will also include acquiring information about the patient's prior medical history, such as any previous abdominal operations or diseases that may resemble appendicitis. Additionally, the doctor will question about the patient's medicines, allergies, and any relevant family history of abdominal disorders.

Laboratory Tests

Laboratory testing may help diagnose appendicitis. The most frequent blood test is a complete blood count (CBC), which looks for symptoms of illness such as an increased white blood cell count. A high white blood cell count, along with an increased amount of neutrophils (a kind of white blood cell), may suggest an inflammatory condition, as is seen in appendicitis.

In rare circumstances, the doctor may prescribe further blood tests, such as a thorough metabolic panel, to evaluate organ function and rule out other possible causes of stomach discomfort.

Imaging Studies (Ultrasound, CT scan)

Imaging tests are useful for verifying the diagnosis of appendicitis and assessing its severity. Ultrasound and computed tomography (CT) scans are two commonly utilized imaging modalities.

Ultrasound is often the first imaging examination conducted, particularly in infants and pregnant women, since it does not need radiation exposure. An ultrasound uses sound waves to produce pictures of the abdomen, enabling the doctor to see the appendix and search for symptoms of inflammation, such as an enlarged, inflamed appendix or fluid surrounding it.

In contrast, a CT scan offers more detailed views of the abdomen and pelvis. It may correctly detect an inflamed or swollen appendix, as well as consequences including abscess development or perforation.

CT scans are especially helpful when the diagnosis is ambiguous or consequences are expected.

Appendicitis is diagnosed using a combination of physical examination, medical history evaluation, laboratory testing, and imaging investigations. These techniques assist healthcare personnel in properly diagnosing appendicitis and determining the best course of therapy for the patient.

CHAPTER 3

Complications Of Appendicitis

Perforation

One of the most dangerous consequences of appendicitis is perforation, which occurs when the appendix ruptures or bursts open. When the appendix becomes inflamed owing to a blockage, pressure builds up within, causing tissue damage and perhaps rupture. Perforation may occur at any stage of appendicitis, although it is more prevalent when treatment is delayed.

Once the appendix perforates, microorganisms from the gut may enter the abdominal cavity, causing infection and inflammation. This might result in serious problems such as peritonitis, which is an infection of the abdominal cavity lining.

Perforation may also cause an abscess, which is a pocket of pus that forms in reaction to the infection.

Perforated appendicitis symptoms may include rapid pain respite followed by increasing symptoms, fever, chills, elevated heart rate, and an overall sense of malaise. If a perforation is detected, rapid surgical intervention is required to clear the abdominal cavity, remove contaminated tissue, and heal the hole.

Abscess Formation

Another dangerous consequence associated with appendicitis is the development of an abscess. An abscess is a small collection of pus that occurs in the abdominal cavity or around the appendix. It usually arises as the body's immune system tries to stop the spread of infection from a ruptured appendix.

An abscess may cause chronic or recurring symptoms including fever, chills, stomach discomfort, and soreness. If an abscess is not treated, it may lead to consequences including intestinal blockage or sepsis. An abscess is generally diagnosed using imaging techniques such as an ultrasound or a CT scan to view the accumulation of pus.

Drainage is commonly used to remove pus from an abscess and reduce pressure on surrounding tissues. This may be accomplished using a treatment known as percutaneous drainage, which involves inserting a needle or catheter into the abscess and draining the fluid using imaging guidance. In some circumstances, surgery may be required to remove the abscess and infected tissue.

Peritonitis

Peritonitis is a dangerous complication caused by an infection that inflames the lining of the abdominal cavity. The spread of germs from a perforated appendix is the most frequent cause, although it may also be caused by a burst abdominal organ or a penetrating injury.

Peritonitis symptoms may include severe stomach discomfort that intensifies with movement or contact, abdominal soreness, bloating, fever, nausea, vomiting, and an increased heart rate. If left untreated, peritonitis may progress to septic shock, a potentially fatal illness marked by dangerously low blood pressure and organ failure.

Peritonitis is normally diagnosed by a physical examination, blood tests to look for symptoms of infection, and imaging procedures like X-rays or CT scans to determine the source of the infection.

Antibiotics to combat the infection, intravenous fluids to keep you hydrated, and surgery to remove the cause of the infection and repair any abdominal cavity damage are typically required for treatment.

In conclusion, complications of appendicitis such as perforation, abscess development, and peritonitis may be dangerous and need immediate medical intervention. Recognizing the signs of these problems and seeking prompt treatment is critical for avoiding more complications and improving results.

CHAPTER 4

Treatment Options

Appendectomy: Surgical Removal Of The Appendix

The main therapy for appendicitis is appendectomy, which involves surgically removing the appendix. It's a method that has been honed over decades to properly treat this problem. When appendicitis is identified, the inflamed appendix is usually removed to avoid rupture and future problems.

An appendectomy involves the surgeon making an incision in the lower right belly, accessing the appendix, and removing it. This may be accomplished by standard open surgery or laparoscopically, depending on the degree of the inflammation and the patient's general condition.

Laparoscopic Vs. Open Surgery

Laparoscopic surgery, often known as minimally invasive surgery, involves making many small incisions in the belly to introduce specialized equipment and a tiny camera. The camera displays a view of the interior organs on a monitor, enabling the surgeon to do the treatment precisely. Laparoscopic appendectomy has various advantages over conventional open surgery, such as smaller incisions, less postoperative discomfort, shorter hospital stays, and faster recovery periods.

In contrast, open surgery entails creating a single bigger incision in the lower right abdomen to provide direct access to the appendix. While it is a more intrusive method than laparoscopy, open surgery may be required in situations of complicated appendicitis or problems during a laparoscopic treatment.

The decision between laparoscopic and open surgery is based on the patient's general health, the severity of the appendicitis, and the surgeon's experience. Both treatments have benefits and drawbacks, and the selection is taken on an individual basis to achieve the best result for the patient.

Antibiotics Therapy

In rare circumstances, especially when the appendix has not burst and the patient's health is stable, antibiotics may be administered instead of surgery. Antibiotic treatment seeks to minimize inflammation and infection in the appendix, enabling it to recover without requiring surgical intervention.

This method is usually reserved for individuals with uncomplicated appendicitis who are regarded as acceptable candidates by their healthcare physician. It's crucial to remember that, although antibiotics may be beneficial in treating mild appendicitis, there is a chance of recurrence, and surgery may still be required in the future.

Antibiotic treatment for appendicitis is often given in a hospital environment, where patients may be carefully watched for evidence of increasing symptoms or complications. It often consists of a course of intravenous antibiotics followed by oral medicines to ensure that the infection is eliminated.

While antibiotic therapy provides a non-surgical treatment option for appendicitis, it is not appropriate for everyone, and the choice to follow this strategy should be taken in conjunction with a healthcare expert. Close monitoring and follow-up care are required to guarantee antibiotic efficacy and handle any possible problems.

CHAPTER 5

Preparing For Surgery

Preoperative Instructions

Before having appendicitis surgery, it is essential to follow specific preoperative guidelines to guarantee a satisfactory outcome. Your surgeon will offer you precise suggestions customized to your unique circumstances, but here are some broad directions you should expect:

First and foremost, adhere to any food limitations prescribed by your healthcare provider. To avoid difficulties during anesthesia, you may need to fast for some time before the operation. Make careful to ask your surgeon about the drugs you should avoid before the surgery since some might raise the risk of bleeding or problems.

In addition to food restrictions, you may be required to undertake preoperative testing, such as blood tests or imaging scans, to evaluate your general health and select the best course of treatment for surgery. Attend all planned visits and follow any extra directions from your healthcare professional.

Another key component of surgical preparation is making arrangements for transportation to and from the hospital. It is not safe to drive yourself home following the surgery since you will most likely be under anesthesia. Arrange for a friend or family member to accompany you to the hospital and then pick you up.

Finally, psychologically prepare for surgery and recuperation. Inform your healthcare professional of any worries or issues you may have, and ask questions to ensure you completely understand what to anticipate.

Having a positive outlook and a support system in place may assist in reducing anxiety and encourage a faster recovery.

Following these preoperative guidelines and collaborating closely with your healthcare team can ensure that you are fully prepared for surgery and increase your chances of a favorable result.

Risks And Benefits

Surgery for appendicitis, like any other surgical operation, has risks and benefits that should be considered before making a choice. Understanding the risks and rewards is critical for making an educated decision regarding your healthcare.

One of the key advantages of surgery for appendicitis is that it may efficiently remove the inflamed appendix, preventing it from rupturing and creating potentially fatal complications such as peritonitis.

By removing the appendix, you may relieve symptoms like stomach pain and fever while also lowering your chance of recurring appendicitis in the future.

However, surgery has inherent hazards, such as anesthesia, infection, bleeding, and injury to adjacent organs or tissues. While these risks are minimal, they must be discussed with your physician and balanced against the possible advantages of surgery.

In addition to the immediate dangers of surgery, it is essential to examine the long-term consequences and problems. While most individuals recover after an appendectomy without incident, others may develop problems such as abdominal adhesions or persistent discomfort.

Finally, the choice to undertake surgery should be made after a full conversation with your healthcare professional, taking into consideration your specific medical history, preferences, and risk factors.

Your surgeon can explain the risks and advantages of appendix surgery and help you make the best choice for your health and well-being.

What To Expect During Hospitalization

When you arrive at the hospital for surgery, you will go through numerous processes to prepare for the operation and ensure your comfort and safety while in the hospital.

First, you will be admitted to the hospital and escorted to the preoperative room, where you will change into a hospital gown and have your vital signs checked. You may also be given intravenous (IV) fluids to ensure that you are properly hydrated before the operation.

Next, you will meet with your surgical team, which will include your surgeon, anesthesiologist, and nursing staff, to go over the specifics of your operation and answer any concerns you may have. Your surgeon will additionally mark the surgical site to ensure that just the appropriate region is operated on.

Before the operation, you will be given an anesthetic to put you to sleep and keep you from experiencing any discomfort throughout it. The kind of anesthetic used will be determined by your unique requirements and the details of your operation, and your anesthesia team will carefully monitor you during the process to guarantee your safety.

During the procedure, your surgeon will create a tiny incision in your belly to access and remove your appendix. In certain circumstances, this may be accomplished using minimally invasive procedures like laparoscopy, which involves making numerous tiny incisions and performing the operation with a camera and specialized equipment.

After the appendix is removed, your surgeon will cover the wound with sutures or surgical staples and apply dressings as necessary. You will then be transferred to a recovery area, where you will gradually awaken from anesthesia under the care of your nursing staff.

After surgery, you will most likely spend a day or two in the hospital to recuperate and avoid problems. During this time, you will be given pain medication as required, and your healthcare team will monitor your progress and offer instructions for postoperative care and follow-up.

Knowing what to anticipate during hospitalization after appendix surgery may help you feel more prepared and confident as you go through this crucial medical operation. Working closely with your healthcare team and following their recommendations may help ensure that your rehabilitation goes smoothly and successfully.

CHAPTER 6

Recovery Process

Postoperative Care

Proper postoperative care is essential for a successful recovery after an appendectomy. Your healthcare team will regularly monitor your condition to ensure it goes as planned. Here's what you may anticipate throughout your postoperative treatment.

Expect regular monitoring of vital indicators like as heart rate, blood pressure, and temperature. This allows healthcare personnel to notice any indicators of issues early on.

Pain Management: Pain is typical after surgery. Your healthcare team will provide pain treatment drugs as required to keep you comfortable.

Please share any discomfort you are having so that your pain management strategy may be adjusted.

Incision Care: Taking care of your surgical incision is critical to preventing infection and promoting recovery. Your healthcare professional will provide you with specific instructions for cleaning and dressing the incision site.

Activity Level: While it is important to relax and allow your body to recover, mild activity and walking may help avoid issues like blood clots. Your healthcare staff will advise you on when it is safe to resume regular activities.

Follow-up visits: You will most likely need to arrange follow-up visits with your healthcare practitioner to assess your progress and remove any stitches or staples.

Pain Management

Pain management is an important part of post-appendectomy therapy. Here's what you should know about dealing with pain following surgery:

Medications: Your doctor will prescribe pain relievers to help you cope with postoperative discomfort. These may include opioids for severe pain and nonsteroidal anti-inflammatory medications (NSAIDs) for lesser discomfort.

Timing: Take your pain meds as prescribed by your healthcare professional. It is critical to keep ahead of the pain by taking your meds on time, rather than waiting until it gets severe.

Side Effects: Be cautious that pain drugs may cause drowsiness, constipation, or nausea. If you suffer any adverse effects, inform your doctor.

 In addition to pharmaceuticals, relaxation methods, deep breathing exercises, and heat treatment may all aid with pain relief.

 Do not be afraid to speak with your healthcare provider about your pain levels and any concerns you may have. They may change your pain management strategy to keep you as comfortable as possible throughout your recovery.

Dietary Guidelines

Proper nutrition is essential in the healing process after an appendectomy. Here are a few dietary tips to follow:

Clear Liquids: During the early phases of recuperation, you may be restricted to clear liquids like water, broth, and apple juice. These drinks reduce dehydration and are gentle on the digestive tract.

Progressive Diet: As your tolerance grows, you may progressively switch to a more substantial diet. Begin with simple, readily digested items like crackers, bread, and applesauce before reintroducing more foods into your diet.

Fiber: Once your digestive system is back to normal, gradually resume eating fiber-rich meals including fruits, vegetables, and whole grains. Fiber helps to avoid constipation, which is common after surgery.

Hydration: Drink lots of water throughout the day. Drink at least eight glasses of water each day and avoid caffeinated and carbonated drinks, since they might irritate the digestive system.

Portion Control: Watch your portion sizes and prevent overeating, particularly in the early stages of recovery. Eating smaller, more frequent meals may benefit your digestive system.

Avoid Certain meals: Some meals may be more difficult to digest or irritate your digestive system during the recuperation period. These may include hot, fatty, and fiber-rich meals.

Consult Your Healthcare physician: If you have any questions or concerns regarding your diet while recovering, please contact your healthcare physician or a qualified dietitian. They may provide individualized advice based on your specific requirements and interests.

CHAPTER 7

Complications After Surgery

Wound Infection

Wound infection is a possible consequence of appendectomy, which is the surgical removal of the appendix. Although appendectomies are usually done using minimally invasive procedures like laparoscopy, there is still a risk of infection at the incision site.

One of the most common causes of wound infection is bacteria entering the incision during or after surgery. Despite rigorous surgical methods and clean circumstances in the operating room, germs may sometimes enter the incision and cause infection. Furthermore, inadequate wound care after surgery might raise the risk of infection.

A wound infection may cause redness, swelling, warmth, and discomfort at the incision site. In certain circumstances, pus may be present. It is critical to regularly examine the incision site after surgery and report any indications of infection to your healthcare physician right once.

Antibiotics are often used to remove the germs that cause wound infections. In certain situations, the incision may have to be opened and drained to remove fluid and debris. Proper wound care, including keeping the area clean and dry, is critical for avoiding future issues.

Wound infection prevention is a top goal both during and after surgery. Surgeons use tight measures to reduce the danger of contamination during the treatment. Patients may lower their risk of infection by carefully following post-operative instructions and keeping the incision site clean and dry.

Adhesive Bowel Obstruction

Adhesive bowel obstruction is a long-term problem that may develop after appendectomy. This problem develops when scar tissue, known as adhesions, grows in the abdomen after surgery and blocks the intestines.

Adhesions may form as a normal part of the healing process after surgery. However, in certain situations, they may become thick and fibrous, resulting in issues including intestinal blockage. Adhesive bowel obstruction symptoms include stomach discomfort, bloating, nausea, vomiting, and constipation.

The risk of sticky bowel obstruction rises with a history of abdominal surgery, several abdominal operations, and particular surgical methods. While laparoscopic appendectomy has a reduced risk of adhesions than open surgery, adhesions may form regardless of surgical method.

Adhesive bowel obstruction is often treated in a hospital setting with supportive treatment such as colon rest, intravenous fluids, and pain medication. In certain circumstances, surgery may be required to remove adhesions and alleviate the blockage.

Preventing sticky bowel obstruction entails reducing the likelihood of adhesion development after surgery. Surgeons utilize procedures like careful tissue manipulation and anti-adhesion barriers to limit the chance of adhesion formation. Despite these precautions, adhesions may still form, especially in individuals who are prone to developing scar tissue.

Recovery Challenges

Patients may face a variety of physical and mental obstacles throughout their recovery after an appendectomy. While appendectomies are regularly done and considered routine, each person's experience and recovery time may vary.

Physical problems during recuperation may include incision site pain, restricted movement, exhaustion, and eating difficulty. To ensure a smooth recovery, patients must strictly adhere to their healthcare provider's recommendations for pain management, activity level, and dietary restrictions.

Emotional issues may also emerge during the healing period, especially if the operation was unexpected or if complications occurred. Patients may suffer anxiety, frustration, or melancholy throughout the rehabilitation process. Patients should talk honestly with their healthcare professionals about any worries or feelings they may be experiencing.

Friends and relatives may provide vital support throughout the rehabilitation process. A robust support system may provide emotional encouragement, help with everyday activities, and company during a potentially difficult period.

Patients should also emphasize self-care throughout recovery, which includes getting enough rest, being hydrated, and using relaxation methods to reduce stress. Engaging in modest physical exercise as tolerated may also help with healing and general well-being.

Overall, although recovery after an appendectomy may be difficult, with good care, support, and patience, most patients should expect to heal completely and return to regular activities within a few weeks.

CHAPTER 8

Prevention Strategies

Lifestyle Modifications

Preventing appendicitis frequently entails making lifestyle changes that minimize the likelihood of acquiring the illness. Maintaining a healthy diet is an important consideration. A diet high in fiber from fruits, vegetables, and whole grains may help encourage regular bowel movements and reduce constipation, which is a risk factor for appendicitis. Additionally, keeping hydrated by drinking enough water may help keep the digestive system running smoothly.

Regular exercise is another key lifestyle element in avoiding appendicitis. Exercise improves bowel regularity and overall digestive health. It also helps to maintain a healthy weight, which is important since obesity has been related to a higher risk of appendicitis.

Furthermore, maintaining proper cleanliness might help avoid infections that could develop into appendicitis. Washing your hands often, particularly before eating and after using the toilet, may help lower the risk of bacterial infection.

Recognizing Early Symptoms

Recognizing the early signs of appendicitis is critical for timely diagnosis and treatment. While the characteristic symptom is abdominal discomfort that begins around the navel and spreads to the lower right side of the abdomen, the presentation varies from person to person.

Other typical symptoms include nausea, vomiting, lack of appetite, and a mild temperature. Some people may also develop abdominal bloating and constipation.

In other circumstances, especially in youngsters and pregnant women, the site of pain might be different or less prominent, making identification more difficult.

It is important to pay attention to any changes in your body and get medical assistance if you develop symptoms that suggest appendicitis. Ignoring or delaying treatment might result in potentially fatal complications such as a burst appendix.

Seeking Prompt Medical Attention

When you have symptoms of appendicitis, get medical assistance right once. Delaying treatment might result in problems like a burst appendix, which can lead to a dangerous infection called peritonitis.

When you arrive at the hospital or clinic, healthcare personnel will do a complete physical examination and may prescribe diagnostic tests such as blood tests, imaging investigations like an ultrasound or CT scan, and potentially a urinalysis to rule out other causes of stomach discomfort.

If appendicitis is suspected, the conventional treatment is surgical removal of the appendix (appendectomy). This treatment is often done laparoscopically, using tiny incisions and a camera to direct the surgeon. In certain circumstances, if the appendix has already burst or there are problems, open surgery may be required.

Most patients recover from surgery without difficulties and can resume regular activities within a few weeks. To ensure a smooth recovery, follow your healthcare provider's post-operative care recommendations.

CHAPTER 9

Faqs About Appendicitis

Can Appendicitis Resolve On Its Own?

The idea that appendicitis would resolve on its own is a frequently asked issue and source of anxiety. While it is true that some instances of appendicitis resolve without intervention, it is important to recognize the dangers associated with waiting for this to occur. Appendicitis occurs when the appendix gets inflamed, which is generally caused by fecal matter obstruction, a foreign substance, or an infection. If left untreated, it might result in serious consequences, such as a burst appendix, which is potentially fatal.

A milder variant of appendicitis known as "chronic appendicitis" may occur with sporadic symptoms that seem to subside on their own before returning later. However, even in these circumstances, the underlying problem remains, and without effective treatment, the danger of consequences continues.

Delaying treatment for appendicitis is perilous because as the inflammation worsens, the appendix may burst, spilling its contents into the abdominal cavity and causing a deadly infection known as peritonitis. Peritonitis may progress to sepsis, a potentially fatal illness in which the body's reaction to infection results in extensive inflammation and organ malfunction.

The essential message is that, although appendicitis symptoms may seem to resolve without medical care, it is not recommended to depend on this. Seeking immediate medical assistance is critical for correctly diagnosing and treating appendicitis before it worsens into a more dangerous disease.

Is Appendicitis Contagious?

Appendicitis is not communicable. It is not caused by germs or viruses that may spread from person to person by direct touch, respiratory droplets, or other infectious disease transmission mechanisms. Instead, appendicitis is caused by a blockage in the appendix, which is often caused by feces, a foreign substance, or infection.

However, it is important to understand that certain diseases or disorders that might cause appendicitis can be communicable. For example, if appendicitis is caused by gastroenteritis (stomach flu) or a sexually transmitted infection (STI) such as chlamydia, the diseases may be infectious. In certain circumstances, the underlying ailment that causes appendicitis may be communicable, but appendicitis is not.

It's also worth noting that, although appendicitis is not infectious, the consequences of untreated appendicitis, such as peritonitis (abdominal cavity infection), may be severe and possibly fatal. As a result, if someone nearby develops appendicitis symptoms, they must seek medical assistance right once to avoid complications.

Can I Prevent Appendicitis?

It is difficult to completely prevent appendicitis since the specific reason is not always evident. However, there are things you may do to possibly minimize your chance of having appendicitis or its consequences.

Maintaining a healthy diet and lifestyle is one potential prevention strategy. According to some studies, eating a high-fiber diet and avoiding processed foods may help prevent appendix obstructions, which may lead to appendicitis.

Eating enough fruits, vegetables, whole grains, and legumes may help maintain a healthy digestive tract and lower the chance of having appendicitis.

Staying hydrated is also beneficial to overall digestive health. Drinking enough water every day may help avoid constipation, which is a major risk factor for appendicitis. Avoiding excessive alcohol and smoke usage may also benefit gut health and lower the incidence of appendicitis.

While there is no sure method to avoid appendicitis, keeping aware of your general health and getting fast medical assistance if you encounter symptoms such as stomach pain, nausea, vomiting, or fever may help diagnose and treat appendicitis early on, lowering the risk of complications. If you have a family history of appendicitis or other risk factors, talking about preventative options with your doctor may be useful.

CHAPTER 10

Living With One Less Appendix

Long-Term Outlook

Patients who have had an appendectomy often express concern about their long-term prospects. The good news is that removing the appendix seldom results in serious long-term health consequences. Most patients heal completely and can resume regular activities within a few weeks.

One of the main worries after surgery is the possibility of infection or problems at the surgical site. However, with good wound care and following post-operative instructions, the chance of problems is reduced. It is critical to keep the incision site clean and dry and to follow any instructions advised by your healthcare practitioner.

Another factor to consider in the long run is the possibility of appendicitis recurrence. While the appendix seldom grows back after removal, there is a tiny risk of developing stump appendicitis, which causes inflammation in the residual piece of the appendix. However, this is very unusual and happens in just a tiny number of instances.

Living without an appendix should not affect one's general health or quality of life. The appendix is not considered necessary for normal body activities, and its removal has no discernible effect on digestion or immunological function. As a result, most individuals may expect to live a healthy and active lifestyle without their appendix.

Resuming Normal Activities

It's natural to desire to go back to normal after having an appendectomy. However, you must allow your body enough time to recuperate before indulging in intense activities or returning to work or school.

You may endure soreness, exhaustion, and restricted movement immediately after surgery. It is important to listen to your body and avoid pushing yourself too hard throughout the recuperation process. Your healthcare physician will normally advise you on when it is okay to gradually increase your exercise level.

Heavy lifting, vigorous exercise, and activities that exert tension on the abdominal muscles should be avoided for several weeks after surgery. Engaging in these activities too soon might raise the risk of problems and slow the healing process.

As you progressively resume regular activities, pay attention to how your body reacts. If you are experiencing chronic pain, swelling, or other troubling symptoms, you should see your healthcare professional. While it is typical to feel some pain throughout the recuperation process, any severe or increasing symptoms should be checked right once.

Follow-Up Care

Following an appendectomy, follow-up treatment is critical to ensuring a smooth recovery and monitoring for any problems. Your healthcare physician will normally arrange a follow-up session to monitor your progress and discuss any concerns you may have.

During the follow-up session, your healthcare practitioner may do a physical examination and examine your symptoms to verify that you are recovering correctly. They may also provide advice on gradually increasing your exercise level and returning to your usual daily routine.

In rare circumstances, further testing or imaging examinations may be necessary to rule out problems or check that the appendix was completely removed during surgery. Your healthcare practitioner will go over any required follow-up tests or treatments and address any questions you may have.

It is important to attend all planned follow-up visits and share any changes in your symptoms or general health with your healthcare practitioner. By being proactive and involved in your post-operative care, you can help guarantee a smooth recovery and long-term health.

CONCLUSION

Finally, appendicitis is a dangerous medical ailment that should be diagnosed and treated as soon as possible to avoid complications. This investigation reveals that appendicitis presents a danger to people of all ages and backgrounds. It might present with a variety of symptoms such as stomach discomfort, nausea, vomiting, and fever, making diagnosis difficult at times. However, with advancements in medical technology and diagnostic tools such as imaging investigations and laboratory testing, healthcare providers can effectively diagnose appendicitis and commence suitable treatment options.

The conventional therapy for appendicitis is surgical removal of the inflamed appendix, sometimes known as an appendectomy. This operation may be done using either standard open surgery or less invasive methods like laparoscopy.

The surgeon's inclination, the patient's condition, and the available resources all influence the surgical strategy chosen.

In addition to surgical intervention, antibiotics may be administered in certain circumstances, especially for uncomplicated appendicitis, or as a precursor to surgery to lower the risk of postoperative complications. However, the efficacy of antibiotic treatment alone in treating appendicitis is still being researched and debated.

Appendicitis complications may be serious, even fatal, if not treated promptly. These include appendix perforation, which results in peritonitis, abscess development, and systemic infection. As a result, early detection and appropriate action are critical to avoiding such negative effects.

In summary, appendicitis is a disorder marked by inflammation of the appendix that requires immediate medical care and treatment. With breakthroughs in healthcare and more public awareness, the prognosis for appendicitis patients has substantially improved. However, continued study is required to improve our knowledge of this disorder and modify treatment techniques for better patient outcomes.

THE END